THE THREE "Es" APPROACH TO A HEALTHY LIFESTYLE

Ed Mahfouz

The Three "Es" Approach to a Healthy Lifestyle by Ed Mahfouz. ISBN 1-58939-228-0 (softcover), 1-58939-229-9 (hardcover).

Library of Congress Number on file with publisher.

Published 2002 by Virtualbookworm.com Publishing, Inc. P.O. Box 9949, College Station, TX 77842, USA

Dedicated to my loving and lovely wife Helen with thanks for your positive outlook, and your help every step of the way.

With love, please accept this as a red rose for you.

TABLE OF CONTENTS

PREFACE

This book was written mainly for us to have fun and to enjoy life. It is designed to put in practice the three "**E**'s" approach as a diet guide to enhance your quality of life: **E**pno, **E**xercise and **E**at. The programs have been carefully prepared to allow you to incorporate them into your daily activities. This book will allow you to pick and choose a program that meets your own particular needs.

This book is an integrated approach to a healthy lifestyle. It is divided into three parts. Part one concentrates on the three "**E**'s" approach and how its application can change our lifestyles. Part two focuses on some practical approaches and lists some examples and strategies of dieting. Finally, part three describes how my wife, Helen, followed the three "**E**'s" approach and the results she enjoyed after following the diet guide.

In this book you will find programs and schedules of diets designed under two major categories. The first category is recommended for people who wish to lose weight. The second category is highly recommended for people who wish to maintain their present weight, but would like to improve their healthy lifestyle by applying the three "**E**'s" approach.

This book is intended to be an approach to a healthy lifestyle. However, I encourage the readers (participants) to preview each part and to consult their doctor should any concern arise. I also encourage readers to review other related materials on diet tips and healthy lifestyles to increase their knowledge and build on the program of activities that is offered here.

Being educated and well-informed about daily activity schedules will help readers to become active participants in pursuing healthy life styles. My ambition and aspiration is to help readers achieve their own personal goals.

Active participation and accurate perseverance in this diet program will ultimately help a person arrive closer to a healthy lifestyle. However, one should keep in mind that all our bodies are built differently and we have unique needs. Therefore, supplementary reading and research on this topic in addition to good medical advice will help each person achieve his or her success.

Finally, I would like to thank my friend Robert Sauder, Ph.D., my friend Jamie Hughson, my son Talal, my niece Tina and my publisher for their excellent editorial guidance in the development of this book and for their many helpful suggestions. I hope this book will capture you enough that you will enjoy a healthy lifestyle. If you start thinking seriously about the three "**E**'s", then I will feel this book was worthwhile. God bless your heart.

PART I

Why am I writing this book?

At the beginning, I never dreamed that I would write a book on health and dieting. But with my wife's insistence that I help her lose weight and stay on her diet, I decided to look deeper into this matter with the hope of giving my wife some support.

In order for me to intensify my research on losing weight, dieting and health, I consulted many resources. There are countless articles available, and numerous materials have been written or published on losing weight and dieting. The Internet alone is full of them, under many titles. Every article and every title has its own merit and its own advantages and disadvantages. It is a good idea for anyone interested in these topics to do some reading.

Together with my own research and the experience of seeing the success of my wife, I felt I could make a positive contribution. But at the outset, I must tell you that I do not claim any diplomas or any recognition on the subject of diet. Nevertheless, I promise to share with you my research, my study, my personal experiences and my knowledge on this subject in the hope it might make a difference for you.

The meaning of the word "DIET"

The word "diet", comes from the Latin word of "*diaeta*"; which can be translated as "way of life". Also the word "diet" can be traced to a Greek origin as in "*diaita*"; which also means a "way of life" or a "regimen". My understanding of the word "diet" is an eating plan that a person follows for a long period of time. In order to make this diet experience successful, I have created a plan that has enjoyable and rewarding outcomes.

My approach

It is my belief that in order to be successful, a person must approach this experience in a holistic way, using all possible angles. The goal is to have a lifelong experience that celebrates aspects of joy and health. Therefore, the effective way to lose weight (if we want to) or an effective way to be healthy for the rest of our lives is based on the three "**E**'s" approach. They are the following: **E**pno, **E**xercise and **E**at.

This first "E" is **E**pno: It is a Greek word that can be translated to English as sleep. Hence, my motto in English is: "*Sleep well, exercise well and eat well*". I take the word 'well' to mean "*balance*" and "*equilibrium*". Furthermore, the number three is a biblical number, and it does bring a spiritual power with it. The second "E" is **E**xercise: Be more active physically. And the third "E" is **E**at: Choose the appropriate diet.

If these three activities (sleep, exercise, and eating) are monitored and observed regularly and for a long period of time, it will become a habitual routine. Afterward, you will notice a significantly positive change in your lifestyle. For example: the level of daily energy will increase. The level of daily production will increase. The look and the enjoyment of life will surely be noticeable. There will also be some other side benefits, like receiving compliments from friends and strangers, and feeling good, positive and confident about one's self. In addition, keep in mind that this will undoubtedly decrease the risk of heart disease or heart attack, and decrease the level of bad cholesterol (LDL) in your body.

As a result, you may notice that the person following the three "**E**'s" approach will release a sense of 'energy' in a room that transmits itself in every direction. Thus, other people in the room can see the 'energy rays'.

Explanation of the three "E's"

The first "**E**" (Epno) stands for sleep. It means the way we take rest. Most of us are familiar with the saying "beauty sleep". As human beings, we learn that our body needs to rest for some time during each day. This rest (sleep) is crucial to us, because our body needs proper rest to be able to perform repair or maintenance. It is essential for our bodies to pause or rest sometime during the day, because it will help us in preparation for the next activity (physical or mental).

I believe that if we do not take care of our body's needs and if we do not properly monitor our time of rest, it may cause unforeseen damage and/or produce unpleasant consequences for us in the future.

We should remember that this book is written under the premise of lifelong enjoyment. Therefore let us examine the sleeping factor. How much time do we need to put aside for this activity? And how can we do it with enjoyment? After all my research and readings, I have come up with a recurring conclusion: scientists and experts do not agree on one specific timetable to accommodate every human being during his/her lifetime. However, we can assume that every individual has his/her own distinct and proper need for sleep daily.

The time of daily sleep can vary from one individual to another. Even for the same individual, this time can also vary depending on certain factors such as the type of activity involved or physical aging. The period of time needed for sleeping every day should be described as a range. For example, 7 to 9 hours of daily sleep is required for an adult of 30 years.

I would like to add here another one of my personal experiences on resting, which I found rewarding and effective: the daily power nap. It has been said that our body is our best doctor. This is true in many cases. So when your body feels fatigued, take 15 minutes of your time to have a "power nap". This should be done once a day, as a daily routine, and on a regular basis. Many studies, research and plain old ordinary folks swear by the power nap, and explain how rewarding it really feels.

Actually, some studies were performed in which companies encouraged their employees to take a 15-minute power nap every day. The results were astounding: there was an immediate increase in production, enjoyment, and agreeable team unity. Furthermore, some of these companies claimed an increase in savings and net profit when losses due to employee illness were considered.

With this technique you will find more daily energy and less daily stress, especially in a competitive and hostile environment. We should all know the negative effects illness or stress has on our body. 'Power naps' will help alleviate this stress.

I recommend that every school board find ways to encourage their students and employees to take daily power naps. I'm sure that they will be impressed with the increase in student achievement. They will be equally impressed with the increase in enjoyment and production shared among the teachers and staff.

It is important that you do some of your own research on daily resting, techniques and scheduling. Sleep time has to be in a quiet place and on comfortable material, away from any external physical stress. Please refer to Appendix B for sleep times. These ranges have been established for a long time. Your task is to choose a table of information that is appropriate for you. Each table is customized for different people and different needs because there are so may factors to consider: age, weight, height, profession, etc. However, because we are focusing on lifestyle in this book, I chose the age factor as a main guide. The reader may still wish to do further research to fulfill his/her own needs for daily rest.

You can help yourself by using the table from Appendix B to organize your own program. After that, you will be on your way to a healthier lifestyle based on the three "**E**'s" approach.

The second "**E**" stands for exercise. There is an old saying: "healthy mind in a healthy body". We all know the importance of an exercise routine to our health. Body exercise is recommended for people of all ages. The benefits of a well-balanced exercise routine are tremendous!

Exercise will likely increase the mobility in your joints, tone your muscles and make you feel good. Also it is a source of relief from our daily work pressures and stress overload. Another side benefit of exercise is that it can enhance our social life and build confidence in our physical and mental abilities. Remember though, physical activity has to be balanced and well-monitored.

I'm not too keen on the saying: "No pain, no gain". On the contrary, I would recommend an immediate stoppage of exercise as soon as the person feels any minor or sharp pain in any part of his/her body. I would also like to recommend that you do some extra reading and research on how to heal a minor injury, care for it and prevent further damage. Consult a doctor or a physiotherapist should pain or injury arise from your physical activity.

To enjoy your exercise, you must establish a routine and a schedule. The general rule says that a person must do an average of no less than 210 minutes of exercise a week. This time is meant for full concentration and focus on the physical activity at hand. This also means that the activity should be evenly spread throughout the week and not condensed into a single day. It can also be balanced within the types of activities.

Always keep in mind that the bottom line is for you to have fun, enjoy yourself and form a long-lasting, healthy lifestyle. Even simple activities can accommodate your needs for exercise. You can do these activities alone or with a group of people.

Some activities bring side benefits like socializing. Examples are walking for the Cancer Society; walking or jogging for the Heart and Stroke Institute; bicycling, walking, swimming, skating or rollerblading to help raise funds for a school or a local charity. In these cases your physical activity is not limited to yourself, but also helps your community in more ways than you think.

The key for you here is to participate and to be physically active. Do not forget to look for these kinds of events in your district. You can also look them up on the Internet. Other activities include joining a local health club, community health center, or a local gym. You may also want to do aerobics or yoga classes, floor exercises and weight training. Therefore, you can also benefit from the advice and the supervision of the local trainers, teachers and leaders.

Other activities that you may wish to participate in can include joining a local team, a neighbor's team or a team from work. This team may hold once a week activities like basketball, hockey, volleyball, baseball, skiing, badminton (goodminton), golfing, rugby, touch football, and ultimate Frisbee. You can enjoy the fun of learning new skills and meeting old and new friends.

You will also benefit from the outdoors and the change of weather. During the summer you can go walking in a park, swimming or even do some mountain climbing. And during the winter, you can go skating or skiing. In this case the long summers and winters become more appealing and less boring. The scenery and the beauty of nature are wonderful to behold.

I suggest that you choose activities that bring you comfort, happiness, and most of all, enjoyment and benefits. Here is a success story about a friend of my wife at the gym. Her name is Susie, and she is in her early forties. She decided to go to the gym with my wife every second day, and do the treadmill for approximately 30 minutes. At the beginning, she found this exercise routine boring and hard. She was complaining to my wife in my presence.

I immediately suggested to Susie that she gradually build on her workout until she reaches her goal. She could go on the treadmill for 10 minutes the first few times, then increase her time on the treadmill by 5 minutes in each of the following two days.

After two weeks of this gradual buildup of exercise time on the treadmill, Susie is now doing 30 minutes every day and having a lot of fun. Furthermore, she is always asking a friend to go with her to the gym, and sometimes I hear her telling others about her recent success. At times, she will challenge other friends to stay on the treadmill for 30 minutes like she does. Therefore, building on your small successes and always keeping a positive attitude will help any person reach his/her goal.

Your physical activity schedule and your weekly exercise must be balanced. Here are some of my personal tips to follow when you are exercising: 1) Stretch before you work out. For better results, exercise should be done when the muscles are warm. 2) Give your muscles a 24-hour break. Especially concentrate on the group of muscles that will be part of your main workout. This 24-hour break is needed to give your body time to heal, repair and maintain itself. It's a rule of thumb that is recommended by many experts in this field. 3) Check the heart rate chart for your age group before, during and after an exercise or a workout.

The third "**E**" stands for eating. Here is an old saying: "we are what we eat". Actually, this activity is the most important one to our survival, because by eating we gather the energy that, among other things, keeps us growing and going. I believe this input of energy has to be observed and balanced in order to achieve a healthy lifestyle. In the following reading I'm not going to impress you with the numbers of calories needed every day, dazzle you with statistics about every food item that exist on Earth, or fascinate you with written studies on the relation between food and genes. I'm going to leave all of that to you to research.

This is what I would like you to learn in order to inform yourself on the whole issue of dieting. I see my role here as shedding some light on the general knowledge of energy and food. I'm going to share with you some examples on how to use this information to build your own balanced diet, which in turn can help you in putting together a healthy lifestyle.

Most of my readings and my research guided me to the following conclusion: food in general is broken down into six major groups. These groupings make it easy for us to follow and to study. They are water, carbohydrates, proteins, fats, minerals and vitamins. Following is general information about each one of those groups, what they are, what they do in our body, and where they can be found in nature!

Water

This makes up the bulk of what we consume. It is approximately 70% of the total mass of our body. Also, 70% of the surface of the Earth is covered with water (what a coincidence!). We need water badly; otherwise we become dehydrated. Water helps our body with lubrication, transportation and absorption. Also, it plays an essential role in our metabolism. We should not forget the role of water in the regulation of our body temperature.

Carbohydrates

Chemically speaking, they are nutrients containing carbon, hydrogen, and oxygen, with the ratio of 2:1 in hydrogen to oxygen. This nutrient includes sugar, starch and cellulose. Carbohydrates provide quick energy to our body. Some of the foods in which it can be found are: rice, cereals, breads, grains, pasta, corn, legumes, and starchy vegetables such as potatoes, squash and yam.

Proteins

From the Greek *Protos,* meaning primary, this nutrient provides primary substance to our body. Chemically speaking, proteins are a group of complex nitrogenous organic compounds. They contain amino acids as their basic structural units. Proteins form the structure of a cell. Whenever cells are damaged, proteins are needed to repair it. Protein is essential, and required to make structures for new cells. Some of the foods in which it can be found are: milk, red meat, poultry, fish, eggs and cheese.

Fats (lipids)

Generally, they are materials insoluble in water. Fats are an excellent source of energy. One gram of fat can provide nearly twice as much energy as one gram of carbohydrate. Fat can help the body to absorb many important vitamins and serves as insulation material under our skin. Also, fat provides protection to some delicate organs and nerves. It is an important component of the cell membrane. Unlike carbohydrates, fats are difficult to digest. Some of the sources in which it can be found are oils, margarine and butter.

Minerals

Minerals are basic elements found in nature. They include calcium, zinc, phosphorus, sulfur, potassium, iron, magnesium, sodium, iodine and chlorine. They help our body to maintain equilibrium in its nutrition. Some minerals, such as phosphorus, carbon and calcium, play an important role in forming teeth and bones. Iron helps red blood cells in their functions. In general, minerals help our body to maintain its normal function. Some of the sources in which they can be found: peas, beans, fruits, vegetables and table salt.

Vitamins

V*ita*, from Latin, means life. (*Amine* also translates to organic compounds; vitamins include amino acid). Vitamins help our body to change (convert) food into energy. Chemically speaking, some vitamins can be soluble in water, like B_1, B_2 and C; others, such as A, D, E, and K, are soluble in lipids. The benefits of vitamins to our body are varied but immense. For example, vitamin K is essential in blood clotting, and vitamin C helps the body to resist infections. Vitamins can be found everywhere and in almost everything that we eat. We get vitamin D from the sun (careful of time under the sun) and vitamin E can be found in grains and vegetable oils…

From what you have read, you can see that we need some nutrients from every group mentioned above in order to keep our body functioning properly. We need a variety of nutrients in a balanced fashion which fits our needs and fulfills our promise of a healthy lifestyle. So let me remind you again: "Sleep well, Exercise well and Eat well." Before I share with you the following table of desired weight, I would like to mention this: desired weight per height is a perceived social image. See tables from Appendix C or D. Those tables are a summary of what most of the experts in this field would agree on.

The Psychological Factor

To arrive at a successful ending, the reader (participant) must make a solid commitment to making their lives more healthy. Mentally, the person has to be prepared, believing that he/she is ready and committed to participate in this exercise and he/she is willing to observe and follow the recommended choices from the three "**E**'s" approach.

To help yourself here, you have to use your willpower. I believe strongly in willpower as the main driving force behind any success.

To will is to opt, to decide and affirm one meaning or alternative from among the many possible ones. To develop willpower, a person has to start making small decisions, one at a time. He/she has to make these decisions with determination. Everybody has enough willpower.

Consider John, my neighbor: he is in his mid-forties—young—and would like to lose 20 pounds. John said to me, "I don't have enough willpower to do it."

Ten years ago, John lost his job. He went back to school for one full year, and at the end he finished his courses with flying colors. He immediately found a new job and is happy with what he accomplished. I reminded John about his willpower when he went back to school and about finishing up his studies, and how much he was dedicated to his study, research, reading books and writing assignments. He never missed a class for the entire year. Moreover, he gave up his bowling night every Thursday just to be in class.

I remember many times when John complained about how hard it was going back to school. Nevertheless, he was determined to stick with his school studies, and that itself required even more willpower. I said to John, "You have loads of willpower."

So we discussed making small and smart decisions, but thinking positively and continuing to build on the positive feedback. For example, John wanted to eat two full-course meals and two snacks a day. Before, he was eating three full-course meals and three snacks a day. So I suggested that he eat three full-course meals and two snacks a day during the first week to start things off. Then I proceeded to tell him to cut down to one snack and three full course meals the following week. Then I suggested that he change one full course meal to a snack the following week. I told him to do this until he reaches his goal.

John followed my suggestions, and he found himself losing weight at an astonishing rate. In addition to his enhanced eating program, John also altered his exercising habits and followed the three "**E**'s" approach. He is currently on his way to a productive and healthy lifestyle.

That's what willpower is all about. When we want something badly enough, willpower will never be a problem!

PART II

This part is divided into three sections. The first section is aimed at people who want to shave off some weight. The second section explains how to maintain a healthy lifestyle with your present, accepted and desired weight. The third section contains a few general recipes that you can enjoy or share with friends.

Section One: Dieting for Losing Weight

15-day trial

Introduction

My approach to weight loss is the following: it should be done gradually, and in moderation. A sudden drop in weight in a short period of time is not a sign of good health. I believe strongly that weight is a perception and a social image. Therefore, your desired weight is a perception of yourself. A weekly average loss of two pounds (approximately one kilogram) is highly recommended if you decide to lose weight. I also recommend that a person should stop following the proposed strategies to lose weight as soon as he/she reached their desired weight (see Appendix C or D).

Once you reach your desired weight, you should follow the advice and strategy given in the second section, starting on page 48. Although losing weight is a difficult process, I believe that it can be done by applying both our mental and physical abilities. You have to be prepared mentally, believe that you can lose weight and remain committed to sticking to the program. In this case, attitude is essential. Moreover, you have to make some physical changes (some people called them sacrifices) in your own eating habits. Sometimes, these changes are not easy. Believe me, there is no such thing as a "quick fix".

To begin, you should take the time to work out a comprehensive diet schedule and program suitable to your needs. Although I'm not a professional dietitian, I am going to share with you my knowledge and my research about dieting. Once again, I recommend that you do more reading and research into your needs. Therefore, the program that you select will be self-based, and you will have sole ownership of it. If you follow these steps, I believe you will achieve good results. You will be in control, and you will improve your knowledge about leading a healthy lifestyle for the rest of your life. Remember, we have to stay in balance with respect to the three "**E**'s".

This weight loss program is intended only for people who are not taking medication and are under a doctor's supervision. I should also add that pregnant women should not follow this program. I advise that you get a medical checkup before you start your program, even if you are not on medication. It is a good opportunity to examine your overall physical condition.

Please keep in mind that you have to be patient and persistent while following this program, and cheating will only inhibit your performance and tarnish the expected results.

Here are some basic processes you have to go through if you want to lose weight:

1. Sit down and discuss the whole program at the beginning
2. Establish a list of rules and conditions to be followed
3. Establish some new habits or kick the old ones out.

4. Monitor and observe your daily progress for fifteen days. Make a journal that includes notes describing your feelings about daily experiences.

Rules and Conditions:

In order to realize success in arriving at your goal, there are some simple rules that must be followed and monitored:

1. You have to make a solid commitment to your program (as long as you are not sick, on medication or under any other restriction) for 15 long and consecutive days.
2. Be positive and keep smiling.
3. Read carefully and understand all the programs and schedules that you build for yourself. I highly recommend that you choose a variety of nutrients in building your program.
4. Build a program which contains ***ONLY TWO MEALS AND TWO SNACKS A DAY!***
5. You can have any nutrients you like, as long as you are not allergic to them. But keep it balanced according to your needs, and follow your program. (Size and quantity must be monitored carefully, and you should follow the recipes)
6. Prepare a checklist after every 15 days to monitor your progress. In this list you can mention things like: feeling hungry, energy level, sleeping habits, etc. (See Appendix E)

HABITS: New and Old

As the saying goes: "We are children of habit." In order to successfully achieve your goals while respecting the rules and conditions, certain habits must be followed:

1. Brush your teeth after every meal.
2. Do not eat any solid foods after brushing your teeth until the next meal. Eat vegetables or fruit snacks instead (mentioned in the schedule).
3. Every time you feel hungry between meals, try to drink a glass of water to relieve your thirst or hunger.
4. Exercise at least four times a week (or an equivalent of 210 min a week, 30 min per day).
5. Eat two major meals a day, one when you wake up in the morning and the other during dinner. Be consistent with the time you choose to eat your dinner (between 6:00 and 7:00 PM). Choose any combination of breakfast and dinner. ***Try to alternate and diversify your choice. Remember, your body needs all six categories of nutrients.***
6. You can have one snack, in the afternoon but it should be limited to only fruits and vegetables. This is for the sole purpose of keeping your stomach busy, thereby eliminating future hunger.

7. Monitor your weight. You should measure your weight at the beginning of the program. Weigh yourself every 3 days at the same time, and with the same scale.
8. Have a "power nap" every day, for between 15 and 30 minutes.
9. Respect and observe your amount of sleep time needed daily. (See Appendix B)

Menu Samples

Following are a few samples of menus that you can choose from. Remember to build your own program according to your needs. Alternating your choice of menu is recommended because it provides a variety of nutrients. The menus are organized under two headings: Breakfast and Dinner. Building your own program depends on your needs and tastes. For better results, choose from the menus below. I assembled these menus carefully. They are a reflection of the readings, research, and studies concerning carbohydrates, calories (input and output) and the body's need for essential nutrients to keep it functioning and healthy.

Breakfast Menu Sample

i) Plain Yogurt/Natural Yogurt (1 cup)
Bread (pita, **1/2** loaf)
Coffee or Tea (1 cup, black)
Apple (1 medium)
Tomato (1 medium)
Water (1 glass)
Skim Milk or 1% low-fat (**1/2** cup)

ii) Cereal (any kind, 1 cup)
Skim milk or 1% low-fat milk (1 cup)
Coffee or Tea (1 cup, black)
Honeydew melon (2 slices, 1" each)
Tomato (1 medium)
Water (1 glass)
Cheese (any kind, 1 slice)

iii) Pancakes (2 medium)
Syrup (1 Tbsp.)
Bacon (2 slices)
Tomato (1 medium)
Skim milk or low-fat 1% (**1/2** cup)
Water (1 glass)

iv) Eggs (1, scrambled)
Skim milk or 1% low-fat milk (**1/2** cup)

Bread (2 slices)
Coffee or Tea (1 cup, black)
Apple (1 medium)
Tomato (1 medium)
Water (1 glass)
Cheese (any kind**, 1/2** slice)

v) Plain Yogurt/Natural Yogurt (1 cup)
Bread (pita, 1 loaf)
Vegetable oil (1 tsp.)
Coffee or Tea (1 cup, black)
Tomato (1 medium)
Water (1 glass)
Skim Milk or 1% low-fat milk (**1/2** cup)

Reminder: If you prefer flavored yogurt, then you must not have fruits. This is a matter of replacement and switching. Also, if you prefer toast, one loaf of pita bread is equivalent to two slices of any kind of toast.

Dinner Menu Sample:

i) Filet of sole (boiled/steamed, 6 oz)
Juice (orange, 1 glass)
Bread (pita, ½ loaf)
Water (1 glass)
Salad (green + vinegar)
Soup broth (1 serving)

ii) Chicken (no skin, 3 drumsticks)
Juice (grapefruit, 1 glass)
Bread (pita, 1 loaf))
Water (1 glass)
Apple (1 medium)
Salad (green + vinegar)
Soup broth (1 serving)

iii) Grilled Steak (lean meat, 6 oz)
Bread (Pita, ½ loaf)
Water (1 glass)
Apple (1 medium)
Soup, vegetable (1 cup)
Cheese (any kind, 1 slice)
Wine (1 glass, red)

iv) Filet of sole (6 oz)
Tabouli (1 serving). See page 59

Bread (pita, ½ loaf)
Soup broth (1 serving)
Wine (white, 1 glass)

v) Chicken (6 oz)
Hommous (1 serving). See page 57
Salad (green)
Wine (red, 1 glass)
Water (1 glass)

vi) Steak (lean meat, 6 oz)
Greek salad (1 serving). See page 58
Soup broth (1 serving)
Water (1 glass)
Wine (red, 1 glass)

vii) **Pasta with chop-chop:**
Pasta (1 cup, fusilli)
Marinara sauce (1/2 cup, heated)
Smoked meat (2 slices, chopped in small pieces)
Juice (grapefruit, 1 cup)
Water (1 glass)
Salad (green)
Soup broth (1 serving)

viii) **Meat balls (Keftedes**, 4 oz or 1 serving). See page 54
Soup broth (1 serving)
Juice (grapefruit, 1 cup)

ix) **Tsatziki** (1 serving). See page 64
Fatoush (1 serving). See page 61
Lentil soup (1 cup). See page 60
Juice (grapefruit, 1 cup)
Water (1 glass)

x) **Stuffed Tomatoes** (1 serving). See page 62
Salad (green + vinegar)
Soup broth (1 serving)
Bread (1 slice)
Juice (orange, 1 cup)
Water (1 glass)
Wine (red, 1 glass)

xi) **Fish & Potato Dish** See page 63
Tabouli See page 59
Juice (grapefruit, 1 cup)
Apple (1 medium)
Water (1 glass)

xii) **Greek Salad** See page 58
Vegetable Soup See page 65
Bread (1 slice)
Juice (orange, 1 cup)
Water (1 glass)
Wine (red, 1 glass)

Snack Menu Sample:

Vegetables and Fruits (have one or two kinds, one piece, at any given snack time). Water (one glass) should be added to every snack, or any other time you feel like it.

NOTES

If you are satisfied (losing an average of two pounds, or one kilogram, a week) with the results after the 15-day trial period, you may like to continue to lose weight until you reach your desired goal. See Appendix C or D. Please do so by following the same pattern and strategy, and repeating the same programs again and again.

Section Two: Maintaining Your Desired Weight

Introduction

Once you arrive at your desired weight or goal, see Appendix C or D. You can start enjoying your new healthy lifestyle by having three meals (breakfast, lunch and dinner) and two snacks a day. You may choose any of the six nutrient groups, but it must be done in moderation and with a balanced program.

Luncheon Menu Sample

i) **Turkey sandwich:** Two slices of turkey (mustard + lettuce + tomato and red onion slices)
Bread (pita, 1 loaf)
Cookies (2 small)
Water (1 glass)
Honeydew melon (2 slices of 1 in. each)
Salad (green + vinegar)
Juice (grapefruit, 1 cup)

Tuna Salad:
ii) Cup canned tuna (packed in water, drained), chopped tomato, onion and celery, shredded carrot and 2
Tbsp. of fat-free Italian dressing.
Juice (orange, 1 cup)

iii) **Pizza a la Pita:**
Spread ½ pita bread with ½ cup fat-free refried beans, ¼ cup salsa and 1 ½ Tbsp. shredded low-fat cheddar cheese. Bake at 375 degrees F until cheese is melted and tortilla is crisp, approximately 12 minutes.
Grapes (1 cup)
Skim milk or 1% low-fat (1cup)

vi) **Greek Lemon Chicken** (1 serving).
See page 56
Bread (pita, ½ loaf)
Apple (1 medium)

v) **Baba Ghannouj** (eggplant, 1 serving)
See page 55
Bread (pita, **1/2** loaf)
Juice (orange, 1 cup)
Tabouli (1 serving). See page 59

vi) **Lentil Soup** (1 serving). See page 60
Salad (green + vinegar)
Juice (grapefruit, 1 cup)
Water (1 glass)

vii) **Tsatziki** (1 serving). See page 64
Hommous (1 serving). See page 57
Salad (green + vinegar)
Juice (grapefruit, 1 cup)
Bread (pita, 1 loaf)
Water (1 glass)

viii) **Vegetable Soup** (1 serving) See page 65
Tabouli (1 serving). See page 59
Apple (1 medium)
Bread (pita, **1/2** loaf)
Juice (orange, 1 cup)

ix) **Hommous** (1 serving). See page 57
Salad (green + vinegar)
Juice (grapefruit, 1 cup)
Bread (pita, 1 loaf)
Water (1 glass)

x) **Fatoosh** (1 serving). See page 61

Broth Soup (1 serving)
Water (1 glass)
Juice (grapefruit, 1 cup)
Watermelon (1 slice, 2 in. thick)

NOTE

If you are underweight according to the tables from Appendix C or D, and your desire is to gain weight, the recommendation is to add another meal (like brunch) during the day until you arrive at your desired weight. In this case, the ideal recommendation is to have four meals and a snack. Then go back and read section two in this book.

Remember to follow the three "**E**'s" approach and to have a variety of nutrients in a balanced fashion.

Section Three: Recipes

Meat Balls (*Keftedes*)

(5 servings)

1 lb ground beef
1 cup onion, chopped
4 tsp. olive oil
¼ cup bread crumbs
1 Tbsp. vinegar
1 Tbsp. oregano
1 Tbsp. salt
1 Tbsp. pepper

In a large bowl, add together all the ingredients and mix well. Cover the large bowl and place in the refrigerator for two hours. After this time, remove it from the fridge and form the mix into 1½-inch balls. Cover a cooking tray with nonstick vegetable spray, such as PAM, then flatten the balls a bit and place them on the tray. Bake at 375 degrees F for about ½ hour.

Baba Ghannouj
(*eggplant appetizer*)
(2 servings)

1 large eggplant
1 clove garlic
1 tsp. salt
2 Tbsp. tahini (sesame seed paste)
¼ cup lemon juice
2 Tbsp. olive oil
1 Tbsp. natural yogurt

Remove stem and wash eggplant; pierce with a fork in 4 – 6 places. Place in baking dish and bake at 350 degrees F for approximately one hour, or until tender. Remove from oven and set aside for a few minutes to cool down. Open eggplant in the center and scoop the contents out, discarding the skin. Place eggplant and remaining ingredients in a food processor and mix for 1 to 2 minutes. Place on a serving plate.

Greek Lemon Chicken

(5 servings)

1 whole chicken (approximately 1 kg)
¼ cup olive oil
¼ cup butter
1 Tbsp. salt
1 Tbsp. pepper
2 lemons
1 tsp. oregano
3 cloves garlic

Wash the chicken. Combine salt, pepper, oregano, garlic and the juice of one lemon; sprinkle liberally inside and on chicken. Place on baking pan, add butter and oil, and squeeze the juice of the second lemon over it. Pour ¼ cup water into the pan. Bake at 350 degrees F for one and a half hours.

Hommous

(4 servings)

1 can chick peas (540 g) (drain liquid)
4 Tbsp. tahini (sesame seed paste)
2 cloves garlic
¼ tsp. salt
¼ cup lemon juice
1 Tbsp. olive oil

Place above ingredients in a food processor and blend for two to three minutes. If it is too thick, add a bit of cold water to your taste. Serve on a platter and sprinkle a bit of paprika on top.

Greek Salad (*a la villagers*)

(6 servings)

2 large tomatoes
1 cucumber
1 onion
10 black olives
¼ cup olive oil
2 Tbsp. lemon
Pinch salt and pepper
½ lb Feta cheese
1 tsp. oregano

Cut the tomatoes in cubes and the cucumber into pieces. Slice the onion. Mix onion, tomatoes, cucumbers, oil, lemon, oregano, olives, salt and pepper in a bowl. Cut the Feta cheese into cubes and toss with the mix.

Tabouli

(4 servings)

2 large bunches parsley
1/3 cup crushed wheat (Burghul)
3 green onions or 1 small onion
2 large tomatoes (diced small)
1 **1/2** tsp. salt
1/3 cup lemon juice
1/3 cup olive oil or vegetable oil

Wash parsley well and drain (you can spin it in a salad spinner). Soak crushed wheat in one cup of water for 5 minutes. Drain well and set aside while preparing other ingredients. Remove stems from parsley and discard. Chop onions fine and add all the ingredients (including diced tomatoes) to a large bowl. Mix well.

Lentil Soup

(6 servings)

1 **1/2** cups lentils
2 cloves of garlic
1 large onion (chopped)
11 cups water
1 lemon
1 Tbsp. olive oil or vegetable oil
Pinch salt and pepper to taste
2 tsp. of tomato paste
1 bay leaf

Place all ingredients except lemon in large saucepan. Cover and cook until lentils are tender. Add a squeeze of lemon juice to taste.

Bread Salad *(Fatoosh)*

(5 servings)

1 head romaine lettuce
2 small pita breads (whole wheat)
1 onion (chopped)
1 cucumber (sliced)
2 tomatoes (diced)
1 clove garlic (crushed)
1 bunch parsley (finely chopped)
1 bunch fresh mint (chopped)
Pinch salt and pepper to taste
2 Tbsp. Sumac herb (optional)
1/3 cup lemon juice to taste
1/4 cup olive oil

Wash and drain lettuce. Tear into bite-size pieces and place in large bowl. Place the pita bread in oven until crisp. Break up into bite-size pieces and add to lettuce in the same bowl. Add all remaining ingredients; toss well.

Stuffed Tomatoes *(Yemistes)*

(4 servings)

8 large tomatoes
3/4 cup rice (washed and drained)
1 lb. beef or lamb (ground)
3 cloves of garlic (chopped)
1 onion (finely chopped)
Pinch salt and pepper to taste
3 Tbsp. of olive oil (optional)
1 cup water

Preheat oven to 375 degree F. Make a 1-inch opening in the stem end of the tomatoes. Hollow out the pulp (save the pulp to add to filling). Add oil to frying pan and sauté meat, garlic and onion until meat changes color but does not fully cook. Mix the cooked meat with rice. Now sauté the mixture again for five minutes. Stuff the tomatoes with the mixture to within ¼ inch of top. Arrange upright in a baking dish. Pour crushed tomatoes over top. Add water to bottom of baking dish. Cover and bake for one hour or until done. NOTE: Potatoes or green peppers may be used instead of tomatoes.

Fish & Potato Dish

(6 servings)

1 lb. fish fillets
4 Tbsp. vegetable oil
2 cloves garlic (crushed)
2 large potatoes
1 tsp. salt
¼ cup fresh lemon juice
1 large carrot
1 large onion
Pinch pepper to taste

Preheat oven to 350 degrees F. Combine oil, garlic, salt and pepper in a baking dish. Add lemon juice. Arrange fish in spice mixture. Peel potato and cut it into ¼ inch slices. Cut carrot into thin strips. Slice onion into thin slices. Arrange all vegetables around the fish. Cover and bake for one hour or until the potatoes are tender.

Tsatziki

(4 to 6 serving)

3 cups plain yogurt
1 cucumber
3 cloves of garlic
1/4 Tbsp. salt
3 tsp. oil
3 tsp. dills (finely chopped)
1 Tbsp. lemon juice

Crush garlic with salt in a bowl. Blend in yogurt, lemon juice and oil. Slice through the length of the cucumber, then chop into thin slices. Add to yogurt mixture. Mix gently. Sprinkle dill over the top for garnish.

Vegetable Soup

(5 Servings)

10 cups water
2 Tbsp. of oil
2 fresh tomatoes
1 cup celery (diced small)
1 cup carrots (diced small)
1 cup fresh green beans
1 cup onion (diced small)
2 Tbsp. tomato paste
2 Tbsp. parsley (finely chopped)
1 cup cauliflower (diced small)
Pinch salt and pepper to taste
1 cup potato (diced small)
Pinch of dried parsley to taste
Pince of dried mint to taste

Cut beans into 1 ***1/2-inch*** *pieces. Place all ingredients in a large saucepan, except parsley and mint. Cover and cook for one hour on medium heat. Remove from heat. Add parsley or mint to taste.*

PART III

Helen's Description of Her Experience in a Healthy Lifestyle

I must mention this at the outset: things that worked for my wife Helen may not work for you. This may be due to factors affecting the diet such as rate of metabolism, genetic factors, choice of food and choice of lifestyle.

Helen described her situation like this: "At first I was skeptical about the 3 **E**'s approach. I never believed that I would lose weight and maintain that desired weight for a long time. Prior to using this diet plan, I tried many weight loss programs. Some programs succeeded at first, but later on I ended up gaining all my weight back and more! When my husband approached me with his new diet plan, I was simply fascinated by it because it captured my attention. I know my husband is a hard worker and when he believes in something, he always gives his best effort into his research."

Helen was working out 4 times a week at the local YMCA/YWCA (every time, her workout was one hour long). She averaged approximately 8.5 hours of sleeping time (including power naps). Helen's weight loss diet program was organized over fifteen days and it was repeated for another fifteen days until she lost 15 pounds.

Helen said: "After a few days I realized I felt really good because I wasn't hungry and I felt more energetic. Even my aerobics class instructor noticed my increase in energy. I was impressed. I lost weight without any hassle. And I was eating the foods I really liked to eat, and I was exercising with added energy. I was sleeping well and everything was much better than before. The changes in my life were incredible."

Helen built a diet program for fifteen consecutive days. Each day had a distinct and balanced diet menu. She repeated these fifteen-day cycles until she arrived at her desired weight.

Says Helen, "The people at my work can't believe the new me".

Now Helen is following the healthy lifestyle program mentioned in section two, starting on page 48, and she is well on her way to enjoying her new and improved life.

Helen's Menus to Lose Weight

DAY ONE:

1	**First major meal:** Yogurt (plain, 1 cup) Oil (1 tsp) Bread (pita, ½ loaf) Coffee (1 cup, no sugar) Tomato (1 medium) Water (1 glass) Skim milk or 1% low-fat (**1/2** cup)
2	**Afternoon Snacks:** Apple (1 medium) Water (1 glass) Carrots (2 slices)
3	**Second major meal:** Fish (boiled/steamed) Filet of sole (6 oz) Juice (orange, 1 glass) Bread (pita, ½ loaf) Water (1 glass) Salad (green + vinegar) Broth soup (1 serving)
4	**Night Snacks**: (No snacks after 10:00 PM) Water (1 glass) Cucumber (1 medium)

DAY TWO:

1	**First major meal:** Cereal (1 cup) Milk (skim, 1 cup) Bread (pita, ½ loaf) Coffee (1 cup, no sugar) Tomato (1 medium) Water (1 glass) Cheese (1 slice, any kind)
2	**Afternoon Snacks:** Watermelon (1 slice, 2") Water (1 glass) Carrots (2 slices)
3	**Second major meal:** *Turkey Sandwich*: Three slices of turkey Bread (pita) Juice (grapefruit, 1 glass) Water (1 glass) Salad (green + vinegar) Broth soup (1 serving)
4	**Night Snacks**:(No snacks after 10:00 PM) Apple (1 medium) Cauliflower (2 pieces)

DAY THREE:

1	**First major meal:** Bagel (1 small) Cream cheese (2 Tbsp.) Coffee (1 cup, no sugar) Tomato (1 medium) Water (1 glass) Skim milk or 1% low-fat (1 cup)
2	**Afternoon Snacks:** Grapes (1 serving) Water (1 glass) Carrots (2 slices)
3	**Second major meal:** Fish (boiled/steamed) Filet of sole (6 oz) Juice (orange, 1 cup) Water (1 glass) Salad (green + vinegar) Broth soup (1 serving)
4	**Night Snacks:** (No snacks after 10:00 PM Apple (1 medium) Cauliflower (2 pieces)

DAY FOUR:

1	**First major meal:** Cereal (1 cup) Skim milk 1% low-fat (1 cup) Coffee (1 cup, no sugar) Apple (1 medium) Tomato (1 medium) Water (1 glass) Cheese (1 slice, any kind)
2	**Afternoon Snacks:** Water (1 glass) Carrots (2 slices) **1/4** honeydew melon
3	**Second major meal:** Grilled steak (6 oz) Glass of juice (grapefruit) Bread (pita, ½ loaf) Water (1 glass) Salad (green + vinegar)
4	**Night Snacks:** (No snacks after 10:00 PM) Orange (1 medium)

DAY FIVE:

1	**First major meal:** Eggs (1 scrambled) Skim milk or 1% low-fat (1 cup) Bread (pita, 1 loaf) Coffee (1 cup, no sugar) Apple (1 medium) Tomato (1 medium) Water (1 glass) Cheese (**1/2** slice, any kind)
2	**Afternoon Snacks:** Water (1 glass) Carrots (2 slices)
3	**Second major meal:** Chicken breast (6 oz) Juice (grapefruit, 1 glass) Bread (pita, ½ loaf) Water (1 glass) Salad (green)
4	**Night Snacks:** (No snacks after 10:00 PM) Cauliflower (2 pieces) Cucumber (1 medium)

DAY SIX:

1	**First major meal:** Yogurt (plain, 1 cup) Bread (pita, ½ loaf)) Coffee (1 cup, no sugar) Apple (1 medium) Tomato (1 medium) Water (1 glass) Skim milk or 1% low-fat (1/2 cup)
2	**Afternoon Snacks:** Banana (1 medium) Water (1 glass)
3	**Second major meal:** Tuna (water, ½ cup) Juice (orange, 1 cup) Bread (pita, 1 loaf) Water (1 glass) Salad (green + vinegar) Broth soup (1 serving)
4	**Night Snacks:** (No snacks after 10:00 PM) Cucumber (1 medium) Water (1 glass)

DAY SEVEN:

1	**First major meal:** English muffin (1) Spreadable fruit or jam (1 ½ tablespoon) Tea (1 cup) Water (one glass) Skim milk or 1% low-fat milk (1 cup)
2	**Afternoon Snacks:** Water (1 glass) Carrots (2 slices)
3	**Second major meal:** *Roast Beef Sandwich*: Two slices of lean roast beef with shredded lettuce, thinly sliced tomato and cucumber Juice (grapefruit, 1 glass) Bread (pita, 1 loaf) Water (1 glass) Broth soup (1 serving)
4	**Night Snacks**: (No snacks after 10:00 PM) Orange (1 medium) Cauliflower (2 pieces)

DAY EIGHT:

1	**First major meal:** Yogurt (plain, 1 cup) Oil (1 tsp) Bread (pita, ½ loaf) Coffee (1 cup, no sugar) Tomato (1 medium) Water (1glass) Skim milk or 1% low-fat (1 cup)
2	**Afternoon Snacks:** Cauliflower (2 pieces) Water (1 glass) Apple (1 medium)
3	**Second major meal:** *Pasta with chop-chop*: Pasta (1 cup, fusilli) Marinara sauce (1/2 cup, heated) Smoked meat (2 slices, chopped in small pieces) Juice (grapefruit, 1 cup) Water (1 glass) Salad (green)
4	**Night Snacks:** (No snacks after 10:00 PM) Watermelon (1 slice, 2") Water (1 glass)

DAY NINE:

1	**First major meal:** Eggs (1 scrambled) Skim milk or 1% low-fat (1 cup) Bread (pita, 1 loaf) Coffee (1 cup, no sugar) Apple (1 medium) Tomato (1 medium) Water (1 glass) Cheese (**1/2** slice, any kind)
2	**Afternoon Snacks:** Orange (one medium) Water (1 glass) Carrots (2 slices)
3	**Second major meal:** *Lentil Soup* (1 serving). See page 60 Juice (orange, 1 glass) Bread (pita, ½ loaf) Water (1 glass) Salad (green + vinegar)
4	**Night Snacks:** (No snacks after 10:00 PM) Water (1 glass) Cucumber (1 medium)

DAY TEN:

1	**First major meal:** Yogurt (plain, 1 cup) Bread (pita, ½ loaf) Coffee (1 cup, no sugar) Tomato (1 medium) Water (1 glass) Skim milk or 1% low-fat (**1/2** cup)
2	**Afternoon Snacks:** Apple (1 medium) Water (1 glass) Carrots (2 slices)
3	**Second major meal:** *Fish & Potato Dish*. See page 63 Bread (pita, 1 loaf) Juice (orange, 1 glass) Water (1 glass)
4	**Night Snacks:** (No snacks after 10:00 PM) Water (1 glass) Cauliflower (2 pieces)

DAY ELEVEN:

1	**First major meal:** Cereal (1 cup) Milk (skim 1 cup) Bread (pita, ½ loaf) Coffee (1 cup, no sugar) Tomato (1 medium) Water (1 glass) Cheese (1 slice, any kind)
2	**Afternoon Snacks:** **1/4** honeydew melon Water (1 glass) Carrots (2 slices)
3	**Second major meal:** Fish (boiled/steamed) Filet of sole (6 oz) Juice (orange, 1 glass) Bread (pita, ½ loaf) Water (1 glass) Salad (green + vinegar) Broth soup (1 serving)
4	**Night Snacks:** (No snacks after 10:00 PM) Water (1 glass) Cucumber (1 medium)

DAY TWELVE:

1	**First major meal:** Yogurt (plain, 1 cup) Oil (1 tsp) Bread (pita, ½ loaf) Coffee (1 cup, no sugar) Tomato (1 medium) Water (1 glass) Skim milk or 1% low-fat (**1/2** cup)
2	**Afternoon Snacks:** Banana (1 medium) Water (1 glass) Carrots (2 slices)
3	**Second major meal:** *Yemistes* (1 serving). See page 62 Juice (orange, 1 glass) Bread (pita, ½ loaf) Water (1 glass) Salad (green + vinegar) Broth soup (1 serving)
4	**Night Snacks**: (No snacks after 10:00 PM) Water (1 glass) Cauliflowers (2 pieces)

DAY THIRTEEN:

1	**First major meal:** Eggs (1 scrambled) Skim or 1% low-fat milk (1 cup) Bread (pita, 1 loaf) Coffee (1 cup, no sugar) Apple (1 medium) Tomato (1 medium) Water (1 glass) Cheese (**1/2** slice, any kind)
2	**Afternoon Snacks:** Apple (one medium) Water (1 glass) Carrots (2 slices)
3	**Second major meal:** Grilled steak (6 oz) Glass of juice (grapefruit) Bread (pita, ½ loaf) Water (1 glass) Salad (green + vinegar)
4	**Night Snacks:** (No snacks after 10:00 PM) Water (1 glass) Watermelon (1 slice, 2")

DAY FOURTEEN:

1	**First major meal:** English muffin (1) Spreadable fruit or jam (1 ½ tablespoon) Tea (1 cup) Water (one glass) Skim or 1% low-fat milk (1 cup)
2	**Afternoon Snacks:** Apple (1 medium) Water (1 glass) Carrots (2 slices)
3	**Second major meal:** Chicken breast (6 oz) Juice (grapefruit, 1 glass) Bread (pita, ½ loaf) Water (1 glass) Salad (green)
4	**Night Snacks:** (No snacks after 10:00 PM) Water (1 glass) Cucumber (1 medium)

DAY FIFTEEN:

1	**First major meal:** Cereal (1 cup) Milk (skim, 1 cup) Bread (pita, ½ loaf) Coffee (1 cup, no sugar) Tomato (1 medium) Water (1 glass) Cheese (1 slice, any kind)
2	**Afternoon Snacks**: Apple (1 medium) Water (1 glass) Carrots (2 slices)
3	**Second major meal:** *Fatoosh* (1 serving). See page 61 Juice (orange, 1 glass) Water (1 glass) Broth soup (1 serving)
4	**Night Snacks**: (No snacks after 10:00 PM) Water (1 glass) Orange (1 medium)

PART IV

WEBSITES

http://www.canoe.ca/health/keepinghealthy.html

Family health guide offers news and articles devoted to dieting, exercise and fitness. Lists associations and has a drop-down menu of diseases.

http://www.chatelaine.com.healthplanner/

View different but continuous articles and topics on health and fitness.

http://www.crhahealth.ab.ca/hlthconn/items/sleeps.htm

Fact sheets covers the different stages of sleep cycles including non-REM and REM, includes general guidelines to help everyone get a good night's sleep.

http://www.dietitians.ca/english/

Comprehensive nutritional resources presented by Dietitians of Canada. Find a meal planner, virtual kitchen and fact sheets on healthy eating.

http://www.fatlossdoctor.com

Discover how to lose up to one pound per day, and keep it off – permanently. Free doctor support.

http://www.hcsc.gc.ca/hppb/nutrition/pube/foodguid/

Shows how to choose items from the four food groups and points out the number of servings needed. Also provides tips on reducing fat intake.

http://www.hc-sc.gc.ca/hppb/paguid/

Initiative from Health Canada that encourages people to adopt more active routines. Applicable in PE classes and on an individual level.

http://www.medbroadcast.com/health_topics/nutrition/index.shtml?

Medbroadcast touches upon three key points to consider when starting a weight loss diet. Read about fat diets and how to start a diet.

http://www.participaction.com/

Bilingual guide provides practical advice, resources and interactive tools to encourage healthy, physically active lifestyles.

http://www.rahul.net/cgi-bin/fatfree/usda.cgi

Offers a search on the nutritive value of various foods from its database, includes links to a site on fat-free foods and USDA food composition data.

http://www.sleepnet.com/

Gives practical advice and contact points for support groups with over 300 accredited treatment centers. Take the sleep test and check out the public sleep forum.

http://www.swdca.org/

Voluntary organization helps sufferers of sleep and waking disorders such as narcolepsy. View brochures, a virtual library, and self-help forum.

http://womencentral.msn.com/fitnesshealth/

View different but continuous articles and topics on health and fitness.

BIBLIOGRAPHY

Anderson, Bob. Stretching. Guidelines and routines on how to stretch. Stretching help keep your muscles flexible. *Shelter Publication Inc*. Bolinas, California. 1980

Barlow, Wilfred. Alexander Technique. Techniques dealing with harmful habits and misuse of the body. *Alfred A. Knopt, Inc*. New York, N.Y. 1973.

Benoit, F. et al. "Changes in body composition during weight reduction in obesity", *Archives of Internal Medicine* 63:4(1965), p.604.

Bragg, Paul, N.D., Ph.D. Healthful eating without confusion: A short book on various diets. *Health Science*. Santa Ana, California. 1975

Council on Food and Nutrition. "A critique of low-carbohydrate ketogenic weight reduction regimens." *Journal of the American Medical Association* 224:10(June 4, 1973), p.1415.

Dement, W.C. and Fisher, C. Experimental interference with the sleep cycle. Canadian Psychiatric Association Journal. August 1963. P.400.

Dugan, A. and the Editors of Consumer Guide. Fitness over 40: A series of guidelines to follow in order to get the best results from the fitness program. *Beekman House*, New York, N.Y. 1984

Ernest, E. et al. " Garlic and blood lipids." *British Medical Journal* 291 (1985), p.139.

Feldenkrais, Moshe. Awareness through movement. Illustrated, easy exercises to improve posture. *Harper and Row*. New York, N.Y. 1977.

Grande, F. "Energy Balance and body composition changes: a critical study of three recent publications." *Annals of Internal Medicine* 68(1968), p.467.

Kasper, H. et al. "Response of body weight to a low carbohydrate, high fat diet in normal and obese subjects." *The American Journal of Clinical Nutrition* 26(1973), p.197.

Kekwick, A. and Pawan, G.L.S., "Calorie intake in relation to body weight changes in the obese." *Lancet* 2:155(1956).

Roberts, P. et al. "Vitamin C and inflammation." *Medical Biology* 62 (1984), p.88.

Saynor, R. "Effects of omega-3 fatty acids on serum lipids." *Lancet* 2(1984), p.696

Solomon, S.J. and King, J.C. "Effect of low zinc intake on carbohydrate and fat metabolism in men." *Federal proc.* 42(1983), p.391.

Stacey, C. L. and DeMartino, M.F. Understanding Human Motivation. An engrossing collection of articles on motivation by several psychologists. *Howard Allen*. Cleveland. 1963.

APPENDIX A: Measurements

Conversion of some of the measurements used in this book, or finding its equivalent

1 m = 100 cm
1 m = 3'3"
1 foot (') = 30.5 cm
1 inch ('') = 2.5 cm

1 kg = 1000 g
1 kg = 40 oz
1 g = 0.04 oz
1 lb = 450 g
1 lb = 16 oz
1 oz = 28 g
1 oz is equivalent to approximately 30 mL

400 degrees F = 204 degrees C
375 degrees F = 191 degrees C
350 degrees F = 177 degrees C

1 slice of cheese is approximately 21 g
1 loaf of bread is approximately 110 g
1 tsp. (teaspoon) is equivalent to 5 mL
1 Tbsp. (tablespoon) is equivalent to 15 mL
1 cup = 250 mL
1 cup is equivalent to approximately 250 mL
1 glass is equivalent to 250 mL

APPENDIX B

Average sleep time per day, by age group

Age Group (Years)	Average sleep time per day (Range)
Newborn (nursling)(0-2)	16-18 hours
Toddlers (2-6)	12-13 hours
Children (7-11)	10-12 hours
Teens (12-19)	9-11 hours
Adults (20-50)	7-9 hours
Seniors (50 +)	8-10 hours

APPENDIX C

My perception of desirable weight for men in pounds according to height

Remember this: "Desired weight per height is a perceived social image". See page 27.

HEIGHT Feet & inches	WEIGHT lbs
5' 1"	110 - 130
5' 2"	113 - 135
5' 3"	116 - 140
5' 4"	120 - 144
5' 5"	125 - 150
5' 6"	128 - 155
5' 7"	132 - 160
5' 8"	137 - 165
5' 9"	142 - 169
5' 10"	147 - 173
5' 11"	150 - 175
6' 0"	153 - 180
6' 1"	157 - 185
6' 2"	160 - 190
6' 3"	164 - 195
6' 4"	167 - 200
6' 5"	170 - 205

APPENDIX D

My perception of desirable weight for women in pounds according to height *Remember this: "Desired weight per height is a perceived social image". See page 27.*

HEIGHT Feet & inches	**WEIGHT** lbs
4' 9"	91 - 110
4' 10"	94 - 115
4' 11"	97 - 120
5' 0"	100 - 125
5' 1"	103 - 128
5' 2"	106 - 130
5' 3"	110 - 135
5' 4"	114 - 140
5' 5"	117 - 142
5' 6"	120 - 147
5' 7"	123 - 150
5' 8"	126 - 152
5' 9"	130 - 155
5' 10"	134 - 160
5' 11"	138 - 165
6' 0"	141 -168
6' 1"	145 - 175

APPENDIX E

CHECKLIST

1.	Did you like the food?
2.	Did you experience any hunger?
3.	How do you rate:
a.	your level of energy?
b.	your sleeping function?
c.	your willpower?
4.	Other comments or observations: ______________________________ ______________________________ ______________________________

About the Author

Ed Mahfouz is a retired secondary school teacher who taught science and mathematics. He is also a former professor who lectured at the Faculty of Education at the University of Ottawa. Mahfouz coached successful athletic teams at the secondary school level, including soccer, badminton (goodminton) and basketball. He is co-founder of Steak & Caesar Restaurant (a fine eatery) in Ottawa.

Mahfouz continues to be an active volunteer in his community and is determined to improve the quality of life amongst his peers. He is the main organizer of a Thanksgiving dinner for the less fortunate, held annually in Ottawa at Sir Guy Carleton S.S. In 20 years of service with his school board, Ed Mahfouz had stunningly kept a perfect attendance record. He attributes this considerably to the three "E's" approach.

Printed in the United States
6561

9 781589 392281